Homem Ice Cream R For Diabetics

Diabetes friendly homemade ice cream recipes

Table Of Contents

Table Of Contents
Terms Of Use Agreement
    Disclaimer
Silky Chocolate Milkshakes
Smoothie Pops
Chocolate Ice Cream
Watermelon-Berry Granita
Lemon-Lavender Frozen Yogurt
Milk Chocolate-Berry Ice Cream
Frozen Raspberry Tart
Triple Chocolate-Hazelnut Frozen Mousse
Layered Frozen Chocolate-Coffee Pops
Ice Cream Finger Sandwiches
Banana Split Ice Cream Pie
Pecan-Maple Sorbet Cups
Frozen Mango-Ginger Cups
Pudding Pops
Tropical Fruit Pops
Watermelon-Tea Snow Cones
Melon-Mango Ice Cream
Golden Pineapple Sorbet
Chocolate Sherbet
Frosty Blackberry-Lemon Ice

Terms Of Use Agreement

Copyright 2015
All Rights Reserved

The author hereby asserts his/her right to be identified as the author of this work in accordance with sections 77 to 78 of the copyright, design and patents act 1988 as well as all other applicable international, federal, state and local laws.

Without limiting the rights under copyright reserved above, no part of this book may be reproduced, stored in or introduced into retrieval system, or transmitted, in any form or by any electronic or mechanical means, without the prior written permission of the copyright owner of this book, except by a reviewer who may quote brief passages.

There are no resale rights included. Anyone re - selling, or using this material in any way other than what is outlined within this book will be prosecuted to the full extend of the law.

Every effort had been made to fulfill requirements with regard to reproducing copyrighted material. The author and the publisher will be glad to certify any omissions at the earliest opportunity.

Disclaimer

The author and the publisher have used their best efforts in preparing this book. The author and the publisher make no representation or warranties with respect to the accuracy, fitness, applicability, or completeness of the contents of this work and specifically disclaim all warranties, including without limitation warranties of fitness for a particular purpose. This work is sold with the understanding that author and the publisher is not engaged in rendering legal, or any other professional services.

The information contained in this book is strictly for educational purposes. Therefore, if you wish to apply ideas contained within this book, you are taking full responsibility for your actions. The author and the publisher disclaim any warranties (express or implied), merchantability, or fitness for any particular purpose.

The Author and The publisher shall in no event be held responsible / liable to any party for any indirect, direct, special, punitive, incidental, or other consequential damages arising directly or indirectly from any use of this material, which is provided 'as is', and without warranties.

The author and the publisher do not warrant the performance, applicability, or effectiveness of any websites and other medias listed or linked to in this publication. All links are for informative purposes only and are not warranted for contents, accuracy, or any other implied or explicit purpose.

Silky Chocolate Milkshakes

Ingredients

- 8 ounces light silken-style tofu (soft or firm)
- 2 tablespoons unsweetened cocoa powder
- 1/2 teaspoon vanilla
- 1 cup light vanilla ice cream
- 1 -1 1/4 cups ice cubes

Directions

- In a blender combine tofu, cocoa powder, sugar, and vanilla.
- Cover and blend until smooth.
- With the motor running, add ice cream in small spoonfuls through the opening in the lid; add ice cubes, one at a time, until smooth and desired consistency.
- Pour into chilled glasses to serve.
- Enjoy!

Smoothie Pops

Ingredients

- 1 6 - ounce carton flavored fat-free yogurt with no-calorie sweetener
- 1 cup fat-free milk
- 2 cups sliced fresh fruit
- 1 cup small ice cubes or crushed ice

Directions

- In a blender, combine yogurt, milk, and fruit.
- Cover and blend until smooth (omit adding ice and blending).
- Pour mixture into 14, 3-ounce ice-pop molds or paper cups.
- If using paper cups, cover each cup with foil.
- Cut a small slit in the center of each foil cover; insert a rounded wooden stick into each pop.
- Freeze pops for 4 to 6 hours or until firm.
- Makes 14 pops.
- Enjoy!

Chocolate Ice Cream

Ingredients

- 3/4 cup sugar
- 1/4 cup unsweetened cocoa powder
- 1 unflavored gelatin
- 4 cups whole milk
- 3 eggs, beaten
- 1 teaspoon vanilla

Directions

- In a large saucepan, combine sugar, cocoa powder, and gelatin. Stir in milk. Cook and stir over medium heat until mixture just starts to boil. Remove from heat.
- Whisk about 1 cup of the hot mixture into beaten eggs; return all to saucepan. Cook and stir for 1 to 2 minutes or until an instant-read thermometer registers 175 degrees F and mixture coats the back of a clean metal spoon.

- Do not boil. Stir in vanilla. Cover and chill for 4 to 24 hours. (Mixture will be thicker after chilling.)
- Transfer the mixture to a 4- or 5-quart ice cream freezer and freeze according to the manufacturer's directions. If desired, ripen.* Makes 1 1/2 quarts, 12 (1/2-cup) servings.
- Enjoy!

Watermelon-Berry Granita

Ingredients

- 3/4 cup water
- 1/3 cup sugar or sugar substitute
- 3 cups seeded watermelon cubes
- 2 cups blueberries and/or halved strawberries

Directions

- In a small saucepan, combine the water and sugar (sugar substitute); bring to boiling, stirring until sugar is dissolved.
- Boil gently, uncovered, for 2 minutes.
- Remove from heat; cool slightly. If using a sugar substitute, combine water and sugar substitute in a small bowl; stir to dissolve.
- Do not heat.
- Meanwhile, in a blender or large food processor, combine watermelon and berries. Cover and blend or process until nearly smooth.
- Add the sugar mixture; blend or process until smooth. Transfer to a 3-quart rectangular

baking dish. Cover and freeze about 2-1/2 hours or until almost solid.
- Remove mixture from freezer. Using a fork, break up the frozen mixture until almost smooth but not melted.
- Cover and freeze for 1 hour more.* Break up the frozen mixture with a fork and serve in paper cups or shallow bowls. Makes 10 (3/4-cup) servings.
- Enjoy!

Lemon-Lavender Frozen Yogurt

Ingredients

- 1/2 cup fat-free half-and-half
- 2 teaspoons dried lavender
- 4 cups vanilla fat-free Greek yogurt
- 2 tablespoons finely shredded lemon peel
- 1/2 cup lemon juice
- 1/3 cup honey

Directions

- In a small saucepan bring fat-free half-and-half just to boiling. Remove from heat; add dried lavender. Let stand 30 minutes.
- In a large bowl combine yogurt, the 2 tablespoons lemon peel, the lemon juice, honey, and the lavender mixture.
- Cover and chill 1 hour.
- Freeze chilled mixture in a 2-quart ice cream freezer according to the manufacturer's directions.

- Serve at once for a softer frozen yogurt. For a firmer mixture, place in an airtight container; freeze 30 to 60 minutes.
- If desired, garnish servings with additional lemon peel, lemon slices and/or fresh lavender sprigs.
- Enjoy!

Milk Chocolate-Berry Ice Cream

Ingredients

- 6 ounces milk chocolate, chopped
- 2 1/2 cups reduced-fat milk (2 percent)
- 1/2 cup sugar or sugar substitute equivalent to 1/2 cup sugar
- 2 eggs, lightly beaten
- 1 teaspoon vanilla
- 1 cup chopped fresh strawberries

Directions

- Reserve 1/4 cup of the chopped chocolate; cover and set aside. In a medium saucepan, stir together the remaining chopped chocolate, the milk, and sugar.
- Cook over medium heat just until boiling, whisking constantly. Whisk about 1/2 cup of the milk mixture into the eggs. Return egg mixture to the remaining milk mixture in saucepan.

- Cook and stir for 1 minute (do not boil). Remove from heat and place saucepan in a large bowl of ice water; stir constantly for 2 minutes.
- Strain through a fine-mesh sieve into a bowl; stir in vanilla. Cover and chill in the refrigerator for 8 to 24 hours.
- Pour chilled mixture into a 1-1/2-quart ice cream freezer. Freeze according to manufacturer's directions.
- Stir in the reserved 1/4 cup chopped chocolate and the strawberries. Transfer mixture to a 2-quart freezer container.
- Cover and freeze for 4 hours before serving. Scoop into small dessert dishes to serve.

Frozen Raspberry Tart

Ingredients

- Nonstick cooking spray
- 1 cup sugar-free dark chocolate cookie crumbs*
- 2 tablespoons butter, melted
- 1 12 - ounce package frozen raspberries, thawed, or 3 cups fresh raspberries
- tablespoons warm water
- 2 tablespoons dried egg whites
- 2/3 cup sugar
- 1/2 cup fresh raspberries, strawberries, and/or blueberries

Directions

- Coat a 9-inch fluted tart pan with a removable bottom with cooking spray; set aside. For crust: In a small bowl, combine the cookie crumbs and melted butter.
- Press the crumb mixture evenly over the bottom of the prepared tart pan. Set aside.

- For filling: Place thawed raspberries in a food processor or blender. Cover and process or blend until smooth.
- Strain through a fine-mesh sieve, pressing with a wooden spoon or rubber spatula to extract as much of the mixture as possible (about 1 cup). Discard the solids.
- In a large bowl, combine the warm water and dried egg whites; stir about 2 minutes or until egg whites dissolve.
- Beat with an electric mixer on medium to high speed for 2 to 3 minutes or until soft peaks form (tips curl).
- Gradually add sugar, 1 tablespoon at a time, beating about 3 minutes more or until stiff and glossy peaks form (tips stand straight).
- Add about one-fourth of the egg white mixture to the raspberry mixture, whisking until smooth. Add the lightened raspberry mixture to the egg white mixture in the bowl.
- Using whisk, gently fold together until no white streaks remain. Pour filling into crust; smooth the top. Cover and freeze for 8 to 24 hours.

- To serve, let stand at room temperature for 10 minutes. Carefully remove the sides of the tart pan. Cut into wedges.
- Garnish with fresh berries. Makes 12 servings (1 wedge per serving)
- Enjoy!

Triple Chocolate-Hazelnut Frozen Mousse

Ingredients

- 1 1/2 8 - ounce package fat-free cream cheese, softened
- 2 ounces dark chocolate or bittersweet chocolate, melted and cooled slightly
- 1 8 - ounce container frozen light whipped dessert topping, thawed
- 2 ounces white baking chocolate (with cocoa butter), melted and cooled slightly
- 2 ounces milk chocolate, melted and cooled slightly
- 3 tablespoons hazelnuts (filberts), toasted and chopped
- 1 ounce dark chocolate or bittersweet chocolate
- 1/2 teaspoon shortening

Directions

- Line an 8x4x2- or 9x5x3-inch loaf pan with heavy foil, extending foil up over the edges of the pan; set pan aside.
- In a medium bowl, beat one-third of the cream cheese with an electric mixer on medium speed for 30 seconds.
- Beat in the 2 ounces melted dark chocolate until smooth. Fold in about one-third of the dessert topping.
- Spread mixture evenly in the prepared pan. Cover and freeze about 30 minutes or just until firm.
- Meanwhile, in another medium bowl, beat half of the remaining cream cheese with an electric mixer on medium speed for 30 seconds. Beat in melted white chocolate until smooth.
- Fold in half of the remaining dessert topping. Spread white chocolate mixture evenly over frozen dark chocolate layer in pan.
- Cover and freeze about 30 minutes or just until firm.
- Meanwhile, place remaining cream cheese in another medium bowl. Beat with an electric mixer on medium speed for 30 seconds. Beat in melted milk chocolate until smooth.

- Fold in the remaining dessert topping. Spread milk chocolate mixture evenly over the frozen white chocolate layer in pan. Sprinkle with hazelnuts. Cover and freeze for 2 to 24 hours.
- To serve, using the edges of the foil, lift the mousse out of the pan. If necessary, let stand at room temperature about 20 minutes to soften slightly. Cut loaf crosswise into 10 pie-shape wedges.
- If desired, melt together dark chocolate and shortening; drizzle over mousse slices.
- Enjoy!

Layered Frozen Chocolate-Coffee Pops

Ingredients

- 1 4-serving-size package fat-free sugar-free reduced-calorie white chocolate instant pudding mix
- 1 1/4 teaspoons instant espresso coffee powder
- 2 cups fat-free milk
- 8 5 - ounces paper or plastic drink cups
- 1/3 cup fat-free sweetened condensed milk
- 1/4 cup unsweetened cocoa powder
- 1/2 teaspoon instant espresso coffee powder
- 1/2 teaspoon vanilla
- 1 1/2 cups water
- 8 flat wooden craft sticks

Directions

- In a medium bowl stir together pudding mix and the 1-1/4 teaspoons espresso powder.

- Add the 2 cups fat-free milk; whisk about 2 minutes or until smooth and thickened.
- Evenly spoon the pudding mixture into the paper cups. Cover and chill while preparing the second layer.
- In a medium bowl whisk together the fat-free sweetened condensed milk, cocoa powder, the 1/2 teaspoon espresso powder, and the vanilla until combined. Whisk in the water until combined.
- Carefully spoon the cocoa powder mixture evenly over the pudding layer in paper cups.
- Cover cups with foil. Cut a slit in the foil over each cup and insert a wooden stick into each slit, pushing the stick down into the mixture in the cup.
- Freeze at least 12 hours or until firm.
- To serve, remove foil and tear away the paper cups or remove pops from plastic cups.
- Enjoy!

Ice Cream Finger Sandwiches

Ingredients

- 1 cup low-fat or light strawberry ice cream
- 12 ladyfingers, split
- 3 ounces bittersweet, semisweet, or milk chocolate, melted
- 1/2 cup flaked coconut, toasted

Directions

- Line a large baking sheet with waxed paper; set aside.
- Spoon ice cream into a small chilled bowl; stir just until ice cream is slightly softened. Working quickly, spread ice cream on the cut sides of half of the ladyfinger halves.
- Top with the remaining ladyfinger halves, cut sides down. Gently press together.
- Dip one end of each sandwich in melted chocolate, using a thin metal spatula or butter knife to spread chocolate over the ice cream.
- Sprinkle with coconut. Place on prepared baking sheet.

- Freeze for 30 minutes before serving.
- Enjoy!

Banana Split Ice Cream Pie

Ingredients

- 1 purchased reduced-fat graham cracker crumb pie shell
- 1 egg white, lightly beaten
- 1 1/2 cups low-fat or light chocolate ice cream, softened
- 1 1/2 cups low-fat or light vanilla ice cream, softened
- 1 large banana, sliced
- 1 cup sliced fresh strawberries
- 2 tablespoons light chocolate-flavor syrup
- 2/3 cup frozen light whipped dessert topping, thawed

Directions

- Preheat oven to 375 degrees F. Brush pie shell with egg white. Bake for 5 minutes. Cool on a wire rack.

- Spread chocolate ice cream in the bottom of the cooled pie shell. Spread vanilla ice cream evenly over chocolate ice cream.
- Cover and freeze for at least 4 hours or up to 1 week.
- To serve, arrange banana and strawberry slices over ice cream layers.
- Drizzle with chocolate syrup.
- Cut into wedges to serve.
- If desired, top each serving with whipped topping.
- Enjoy!

Pecan-Maple Sorbet Cups

Ingredients

- 2 egg whites
- 1/2 cup ground pecans
- 3 tablespoons butter, melted
- 1/4 teaspoon maple flavoring
- sugar substitute equal to 1/2 cup sugar
- 1/2 cup all-purpose flour
- Nonstick cooking spray
- 3 cups desired flavor sorbet
- Fresh mint leaves

Directions

- In a medium bowl, let egg whites stand at room temperature for 30 minutes.
- Preheat oven to 375 degrees F. Line large cookie sheets with foil or parchment paper. If using foil, lightly grease foil; set aside. In a small bowl, combine ground pecans, butter, and maple flavoring; set aside.

- Beat egg whites with an electric mixer on medium speed until soft peaks form (tips curl). Gradually add sugar, beating on high speed until stiff peaks form (tips stand straight). Fold in about half of the flour. Gently stir in pecan mixture. Fold in the remaining flour until thoroughly combined.
- For each tuile: Drop two rounded measuring tablespoons of the batter onto prepared cookie sheets; leave 4 inches between mounds (place only two or three mounds on each baking sheet). Using the back of a spoon, spread each mound into a 4-inch circle. If necessary, coat the back of the spoon with nonstick cooking spray to prevent sticking.
- Bake for 5 to 7 minutes or until tuiles are golden brown around edges and centers are lightly browned. Using a wide spatula, immediately remove the tuiles and gently press each warm tuile into a 3-1/2-inch (jumbo) muffin cup, pleating sides as needed to form a cup. (Or wrap each warm tulle around the bottom of a 2-1/2-inch muffin cup, pleating sides as needed to form a cup.)

- Cool tuiles until they hold their shape. Carefully remove from muffin cups. Cool completely on a wire rack.
- To serve, using a small ice cream scoop, scoop sorbet into tuile cups.
- Garnish with mint leaves.
- Enjoy!

Frozen Mango-Ginger Cups

Ingredients

- 2 mangoes, seeded, peeled, and cut up
- 1 8 - ounce tub light cream cheese
- 1 6 - ounce carton low-fat peach yogurt
- 1/2 teaspoon ground ginger
- 12 gingersnaps, crushed
- 3/4 cup frozen light whipped dessert topping, thawed
- 1/2 of a medium mango, cut into thin bite-size slivers

Directions

- In a food processor or blender, combine cut-up mango, cream cheese, yogurt, and ground ginger. Cover and process or blend until very smooth.
- Divide crushed gingersnaps evenly among sixteen 2-ounce disposable shot glasses or regular shot glasses. Carefully spoon in mango mixture.
- Freeze about 1 hour or just until firm.

- Before serving, let stand at room temperature for 10 minutes .
- To serve, spoon dessert topping on top of the mango mixture in glasses. Top with mango slivers.
- Enjoy!

Pudding Pops

Ingredients

- 1 4-serving-size pkg. sugar-free instant chocolate or chocolate fudge pudding mix
- 2 cups fat-free milk
- 1 4-serving-size pkg. sugar-free instant banana cream
- 2 cups fat-free milk

Directions

- Place sixteen 3-ounce disposable plastic drink cups in a 1392-inch baking pan; set aside.
- Put the chocolate pudding mix into a medium mixing bowl. Add 2 cups milk. Use a wire whisk or rotary beater to beat the pudding for 2 minutes or until well mixed. Spoon about 2 tablespoons pudding into each cup. Cover cups with a piece of foil. Freeze for 1 hour.
- Place desired flavor pudding mix in another medium bowl. Add 2 cups milk. Use a wire whisk

or rotary beater to beat the pudding for 2 minutes or until well mixed.
- Remove pudding-filled cups from freezer; uncover. Spoon 2 tablespoons of second flavor of pudding over frozen pudding in cups.
- Cover each cup with foil. Make a small hole in center of foil with the sharp knife. Push a wooden stick through the hole and into the top layer of pudding in the cup. Put the baking pan in the freezer. Freeze for 4 to 6 hours or until pudding pops are firm.
- Remove from freezer. Let stand for 15 to 20 minutes before serving.
- Remove pudding pops from the cups.
- Enjoy!

Tropical Fruit Pops

Ingredients

- 2 cups chopped mango (about 2 large)
- 1 8 - ounce can crushed pineapple (juice pack)
- 1 medium banana, sliced
- 1/4 cup frozen orange juice concentrate, thawed
- 1/4 teaspoon ground ginger

Directions

- In a blender or food processor, mix mango, undrained pineapple, banana, orange juice concentrate, and ginger.
- Cover and blend until smooth.
- Pour the fruit mixture into 12 compartments of freezer pop molds.
- Freeze for 3 to 4 hours or until firm.
- Enjoy!

Watermelon-Tea Snow Cones

Ingredients

- 2/3 cup water
- 1/3 cup lightly packed fresh mint leaves or 2 small sprigs fresh rosemary
- 3 bags Red Zinger® tea
- sugar substitute equal to 3 tablespoons sugar
- 2 cups seeded, cubed watermelon
- 3 cups ice cubes

Directions

- In a small saucepan, bring the water to boiling; add mint or rosemary. Simmer, uncovered, for 2 minutes. Remove from heat. Add tea bags; cover and let steep for 4 minutes.
- Strain mixture through a sieve, pressing tea bags to remove all liquid; discard tea bags and mint or rosemary.

- Let tea stand about 30 minutes or until cooled to room temperature. Add sugar, stirring until dissolved.
- Meanwhile, place watermelon in blender. Cover and blend until smooth
- Add pureed watermelon to the tea mixture.
- Cover and chill for 4 hours to 3 days.
- Place watermelon mixture in blender.
- With blender running, add ice cubes, one at a time, through the hole in the lid; blend until the mixture is slushy and almost spoonable.
- Enjoy!

Melon-Mango Ice Cream

Ingredients

- 2 cups whole milk
- 2 cups buttermilk
- 2 cups fat-free half-and-half
- sugar substitute equal to 1 cup sugar
- 1 tablespoon vanilla
- 1 1/2 cups chopped cantaloupe
- 1 1/2 cups chopped mango

Directions

- In a large bowl, combine milk, buttermilk, fat-free half-and-half, sugar, and vanilla. Stir to dissolve sugar.
- In a blender or food processor, combine cantaloupe and mango. Cover and blend or process until smooth.
- Stir pureed fruit into milk mixture. Freeze in a 4- to 5-quart ice cream freezer according to the manufacturer's directions.
- Enjoy!

Golden Pineapple Sorbet

Ingredients

- 1 large whole fresh pineapple
- 1/4 cup fresh lime juice
- sugar substitute equal to 1/4 cup of sugar

Directions

- Halve pineapple lengthwise; remove fruit. Remove and discard pineapple core. Chop pineapple.
- Place chopped pineapple in a blender container with lime juice and sugar; cover. Blend for 2 minutes or until mixture is completely smooth.
- Press through a strainer; you should have about 3 cups puree.
- Transfer mixture to a 2-quart ice cream freezer; freeze according to manufacturer's directions.
- Allow to ripen for 4 hours.
- Freeze.
- To serve, scoop into chilled dessert dishes or frozen pineapple shells.

- Enjoy!

Chocolate Sherbet

Ingredients

- 6 -7 ounces 60-percent-cacao chocolate
- 2 cups water
- sugar substitute equal to 2/3 cup sugar
- 1/2 cup whipping cream
- 1 teaspoon vanilla

Directions

- In a medium saucepan stir together chopped chocolate, sugar substitute, water, and whipping cream.
- Bring to boiling, whisking constantly. Boil gently for 1 minute. Remove from heat and stir in vanilla.
- Cover and chill overnight.
- Freeze mixture in a 1-quart ice cream freezer according to manufacturer's directions.
- Ripen in freezer before serving. To serve, scoop into small glasses or dishes.
- Enjoy!

Frosty Blackberry-Lemon Ice

Ingredients

- 1 cup water
- sugar substitute equal to 1/2 cup sugar
- 4 cups fresh blackberries
- 1/4 cup fresh lemon juice
- 2 tablespoons finely shredded lemon peel

Directions

- In a medium saucepan combine water and sugar; bring to boiling, stirring frequently.
- Boil gently, uncovered, for 2 minutes.
- Remove from heat and cool slightly.
- In a blender or food processor combine blackberries, the warm syrup mixture, and lemon juice.
- Cover and blend or process until almost smooth. Strain mixture through a fine mesh sieve, discarding seeds. Stir in 1 teaspoon of the lemon peel.

- Transfer the mixture to a 3-quart rectangular baking dish or a 13x9x2-inch baking pan.
- Place in the freezer, uncovered, for 1-1/2 hours or until almost solid.
- Remove berry ice from freezer. Using a fork, break up the ice into a somewhat smooth mixture.
- Freeze 1 hour more.
- Enjoy!